CHICKPEA CANCER CURE

How to Stimulate Your Immune System and Get Well

CHICKPEA CANCER CURE

How to Stimulate Your Immune System and Get Well

George E. Ashkar, Ph.D.
(Interpreted by Bonnie O'Sullivan)

DEDICATION

Welcome to Cancer Cure,

I am GEORGE E. ASHKAR, Ph.D. I dedicate this book to my beloved wife Angel who tirelessly encouraged me to finish and publish it.

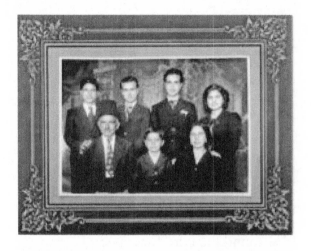

Ashkar family in 1937 Beirut, Lebanon

I was five years old when I promised to find a cure for cancer.

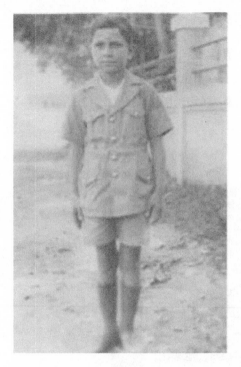

George E. Ashkar, 1943 Beirut, Lebanon

At the age of 12, I found the cure for cancer. I
developed Neutral Infection Absorption (NIA) Method

Foreword

Since 1900 oncologist researchers and oncologist practitioners have never tried to cure cancer, they sought to eliminate cancer cells, which are the victims and not the problem, leaving carcinogens, which are the cause of cancer, in the body to start cancer again and again until the victim dies. If they cure cancer, they will lose their jobs and income. In this book, I recommend my Neutral Infection Absorption (NIA) method which can eliminate carcinogens as well as cancer cells. The recuperation is 100% with no recurrences. This book is designed for the general public to be used as self-service, and for medical professionals. It is priceless information about cancer.

Table of Contents

Invention and Development of Neutral Infection (NIA) Method

In 1936 my uncle Naum Rezkalla Sayegh got stomach cancer in Aleppo, Syria where he was living. He was admitted to the Medical School of the American University of Beirut, AUB, for cancer treatment but he died in few days. I was distraught, and I decided to find a cure for cancer no matter what.

In 1943 my older brother Sarkis went to Tunisia to work in a machine shop of the French army. It was a war zone, and my mother worried about his life because there was an ongoing active war there at that time. Because of that, my mother got Rheumatism. She visited many doctors to find a cure, but it was in vain. No one had a cure for her illness.

As a last resort, we visited our countryman, Doctor Professor Yenicomshlian. He was working at the Medical School of the American University of Beirut, AUB. He also gave us no hope of a cure for my mother's Rheumatism, but he gave her some advice: "Keep warm and dry." And then he added: "Something in the blood is causing that illness, but we do not know what it is or how to get rid of it." His theory on the cause of Rheumatism gave me the idea that illness-causing chemicals should not be in the blood and I began looking and trying to find ways to get them out of the body to cure the illness.

1

One day I was playing with my friends in our backyard, and my mother called me and asked me to prepare yogurt. I was the yogurt maker of our family. I had to boil the milk, let it cool, and then mix in a couple of spoonfuls of yogurt as a yeast to prepare the yogurt. To make it fast and go back to play, I increased the heat to boil the milk faster, and at the end, I noticed the milk had burned and smelled burnt. I had no choice but to continue to make the yogurt with burned milk and return to continue the game.

The next day I woke up early to taste the yogurt, it tasted like burnt milk. A few hours later my mother asked me if the yogurt was ready and I said "Yes" and we went to taste it. First, my mother tasted it, and I was afraid she would complain about the burnt taste, but to the contrary, she praised me as a good yogurt maker. I couldn't believe it.

When it was my turn to taste it, I was surprised that the yogurt was excellent. I tried to find an explanation of what had happened. First, I tried tasting it from the surface of the yogurt. It was perfect. Then, I sampled it from the bottom of the yogurt, and it was bad. It smelled and tasted burnt. To be sure, I tried tasting it again. First from the surface of the yogurt where the watery part of the yogurt had drained off, and it tasted perfect. Then I tried tasting it from the bottom of the yogurt with the watery part still there. It tasted and smelled bad, so I established that all the burned milk was dissolved in the watery part of the milk.

I came to the conclusion that burned milk and chemicals are dissolved in the watery part of the milk. This discovery gave me the idea that disease-causing particles and chemicals in the body should be in the watery part of the blood, so my conclusion was: to get rid of chemicals and particles, which are causing illnesses, I have to clean up the watery part of the blood to cure diseases.

As I was looking for ways to clean up the watery part of the blood from disease-causing chemicals, I remembered if the skin is burned it creates a blister full of serum, the watery part of the blood, and draining the water from the blister will help get rid of the chemicals. Therefore, by cutting the dead skin off the blister and draining the water from it, you will help the body eliminate chemicals.

I decided to test my idea on my mother to cure her Rheumatism illness. I had to make a blister. The only way to make a blister was to burn the skin, and in those days a cigarette would do that, but I did not want to risk burning my mother's skin in that way to make a blister. My mother took the initiative and made the blister by burning the skin on her leg with a cigarette. I was surprised when I saw my mother burning her skin without hesitation. I figured that the pain of

Rheumatism must be worse than the pain of burning the skin. The blister was ready, and I had to cut the dead skin off to empty the serum it contained, so I did. When the serum poured out of the blister, my mother told me she felt some relief of her pain. That was the first sign that the treatment would work.

One blister drained a negligent amount of serum, but I needed a large amount. I knew from my kitchen experience that before cooking beans and chickpeas, we soaked them in water overnight to help them cook faster because beans and chickpeas have the ability to absorb water and that makes cooking them much easier. I put a dry bean on the wound to absorb the serum continuously, but that did not happen and the wound healed.

The next time I decided to put a chickpea on the wound and this time it worked perfectly. The chickpea started to absorb the serum continuously until it got saturated, and when it stopped, because of saturation, I replaced the saturated chickpea with another dry one and in this way drainage never stopped.

Establishing a continuous flow of serum guarantees the removal of all disease-causing chemicals from the body and prevents the wound from getting infected since the flow of the serum is out of the body, so infection has no chance to get in the body, which is very important in preventing the wound from getting infected during many months of treatment.

One day I was eating garlic with bread and playing in our backyard with my friends. I finished the bread but still had a piece of garlic I did not want to throw away, so I kept the garlic in my palm until the end of the game. I saved the garlic to eat later.

When I woke up the next morning, I noticed a blister in my hand in the same area where I was holding the garlic. That gave me the idea to use garlic to make a blister which is more humane than using a cigarette to burn the skin to make a blister.

Using this method in 1943 for six months my mother's Rheumatism was cured completely and never came back during her lifetime, she died in 1970 of natural causes.

This is the way my Neutral Infection Absorption (NIA) method was developed, completed and tested and was ready to be used for all types of Rheumatoid Arthritic related diseases.

In 1960 my wife developed Rheumatoid Arthritis. I immediately used my NIA method to cure her illness, and after six months of treatment, her Rheumatoid Arthritis was cured completely and never came back during her lifetime. She was the second person to be treated by my NIA method. She died December 1, 2007.

Definition of Cancer

The mechanism for the development of cancer is the presence of two agents: Initiators and Promoters. One initiator and one promoter must be present to cause cancer.

An initiator can be a particle (a minute portion of matter) or a chemical (asbestos, food preservatives, fertilizers, pesticides, carbon dust, and other chemicals in the environment).

To start to develop cancer, the initiator has to reach a critical concentration in the body, which, in a normal situation, took 10 to 15 years in the year 2000.

A promoter is a piece of a destroyed cell caused as a natural byproduct of the body's emotional reaction to stress such as fear, worry, a tragedy in the family, or caused artificially by x-rays, radiation, chemotherapies, radioactive materials and finally microorganisms capable of destroying the body's cells.

According to this definition, cure or prevention of cancer could be achieved only by physically removing initiators from the body.

There are two groups of diseases. The first group is initiated by living microorganisms like bacteria and viruses. In this group, diseases are transferable from one person to another by physical contact or by air (venereal disease, flu, etc.). These diseases are successfully cured by using antibiotics in addition to the body's defense system.

The second group of diseases is caused by particles and chemicals (asbestos, food preservatives, etc.). These diseases are not transferable by contact or air. The body's defense system is not designed to fight these kinds of chemical infections. Moreover, medicine cannot eliminate these particles and chemicals; therefore these diseases are not curable by medicine. The only way to cure them is to remove the disease-causing particles and chemicals from the body physically. That is probably the reason there has been no remarkable success during the past century in curing this group of diseases by using drugs, despite enormous success in science and technology.

Surgery, which is the only officially accepted method to cure cancer, physically removes diseased cells and part of the disease-causing particles from localized parts of the body. That is not enough because all disease-causing particles cannot be removed by surgery since they are also in the bloodstream and lymph system circulating all over the body. Some will remain and cause disease again and again particularly when cancer has already spread all over the body.

Cure for Cancer

In 1980 I decided to start research in the field of cancer to find ways to cure that illness. First, I needed professional advice from experts, so I asked a doctor if he knew what cancer is. He said no. Then I asked if he has a cure for cancer. He said no. Then I asked what kind of specialist he is. He said he is an expert oncologist. I was surprised to hear that one could be an expert oncologist if he does not know what cancer is and to have no cure for cancer. To find out the qualifications of the doctor I asked another couple of questions: Why does cancer not have symptoms? He said he did not know. Then I asked why every organ in the body gets cancer except the heart? He said he did not know. I could not understand what he knew except writing fat bills.

I confronted surprise after surprise. First I found that cancer is not a medical problem because it is not a viral or bacterial disease. Instead, it is a chemical disease. Second, I found that oncologists, since 1900, have been trying to eliminate cancerous cells, which are the victims of carcinogens, not the problem, and leaving the carcinogens, which are the problem, in the body to start cancer again and again, which oncologists call a surprising recurrence.

I studied the entire phenomenon happening to people who have cancer, and I suggested a mechanism for the development of cancer, which correctly explained what cancer is when it happens, how it happens, why it happens, where it happens, and how to cure and prevent it from happening.

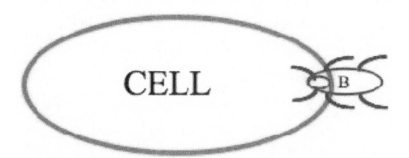

Figure 1. Infected Cell

Definition of Disease

What is a disease? First, I'd like to tell you about viral and bacterial diseases. These diseases start when bacteria or viruses invade the human body and start to damage healthy body cells. (See Figure 1.)

The way disease is caused by bacteria and viruses is that they both use our cells as nutrients to multiply themselves. After enough cells are destroyed, we feel the symptoms of the disease.

Bacteria and viruses give us a type of disease, and damaged cells give us a symptom of the disease. Since bacteria and viruses are living microorganisms, we can use medicine to kill them and cure the disease.

Therefore, if we eliminate the bacteria and viruses, we cure the disease.

However, if we only eliminated the damaged cells, we would only eliminate the symptoms of the disease, not the disease itself and the disease would not be cured since the bacteria and viruses would still be in the body and would continue causing the disease.

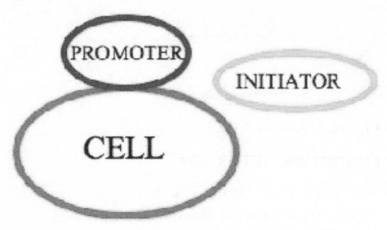

Figure 2. Cancerous Cell

Cancer is different. (See Figure 2.) It is not a viral or bacterial disease; it is a health problem caused by chemicals used in the food industry; therefore it is not a medical problem it is a physics problem. Cancer is a chemical disease and is caused by carcinogens (medical professionals call chemicals "carcinogens," and a carcinogen means "cancer producer").

To turn a healthy cell into a cancerous cell, we need a promoter. When a healthy cell and a promoter become fused together, the body cell becomes cancerous. The problem is a healthy cell and a promoter cannot fuse together by themselves, so here comes a carcinogen to help them fuse together by initiating a chemical reaction between them. Because of its role in initiating a chemical reaction between them I renamed the carcinogen the initiator.

The above process is the only model of how cancerous cells are created; no other model satisfies all the aspects of cancerous cells.

As in the case of viral and bacterial diseases, we have to eliminate the cause of the disease to cure it. In the case of cancer, the cause of the disease is carcinogens, so we have to eliminate carcinogens to cure cancer. Unfortunately, all over the world "Expert Oncologists" since 1900 have been trying to eliminate cancerous cells, which eliminates only the symptoms of the disease, not the problem, and leaves the carcinogens inside the body to start cancer again and again until the victim dies.

Cancer cells are not killing people. No matter how many cancer cells are in the body, a person will not die from cancer. People do not die because of too many cancer cells. Instead, they die because too many healthy cells have become cancerous and too few healthy cells are left in their vital organs to sustain normal function to keep them alive. The main vital organs are lungs, liver, pancreas, stomach, kidneys, and brain. People can survive with cancer in organs that are not vital, even if they are removed, such as breast, uterus, vagina, ovaries, prostate or testicles.

The Mechanism Development of Cancer

The initiator (carcinogen): The mechanism of the development of cancer is very clear and very precise and of course very interesting. To start cancer in the human body, you first need carcinogens or "cancer-causing chemicals." An initiator could be all kinds of chemicals existing in food, such as food processing chemicals, food preservatives, fertilizers, pesticides, asbestos, etc. Different chemicals cause different non-viral, non-bacterial diseases such as cancer, leukemia, rheumatoid arthritis, rheumatism, asthma, lupus, emphysema, bronchitis, etc.

To start to develop cancer the following conditions must be met; in the body there must be a promoter (a piece of a destroyed cell caused by the body's emotional reaction to stress such as fear, worry, a tragedy in the family, or caused artificially as by x--rays, radiation, chemotherapies, radioactive materials and finally microorganisms capable of destroying the body's cells) and a certain critical concentration of carcinogens (the initiator), below which the initiation will not succeed. When the initiator chemically fuses (connects) a healthy cell to a piece of a destroyed cell, cancer is created. (See explanation below.)

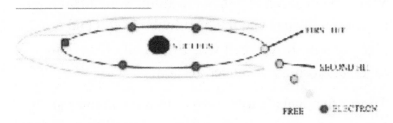

Figure 3. Activation of the cell

Initiation

To initiate the reaction between a healthy body cell and the promoter (a piece of a destroyed cell) and create a cancerous cell, the carcinogen (the initiator) must create an active center on the surface of the cell by pulling out one electron. (See Figure 3.)

When the initiator hits the cell and moves one electron from its orbit to a higher orbit, it immediately needs a second hit to move the electron completely out of the atom to create an active center. Therefore, a critical concentration is needed to guarantee the second hit before the electron returns to its original orbit.

If the number of carcinogens is less than a critical concentration, then the electron will return to its original orbit before the second hit of the electron occurs, therefore the active center will not be created and the chemical reaction between the body cell and the piece of destroyed cell will not happen and no cancer will be created.

When the electron is out of the atom, a chemical reaction will start and the healthy body cell and the piece of a destroyed cell will chemically fuse (join together) forming a cancerous cell.

These chemicals (carcinogens) dissolve mainly in the lymph and will accumulate for years until they reach a certain critical concentration. This accumulation could take many years to reach from zero to a critical concentration. In the following "Note" you can see how the years of accumulation has changed during the past half-century.

Note: Years needed to reach critical concentration of chemicals (carcinogens) was:

In 1950 between 40-50 years
In 1960 between 30-40 years
In 1970 between 20-30 years
In 1980 between 15-20 years
In 1990 between 10-15 years and the time needed is continuing to shrink; it is the result of intensive use of chemicals in the food industry.

These types of diseases (cancer, arthritis, lupus, leukemia, asthma, colitis, etc.), which result from the accumulation of carcinogens in the plasma, according to medical professionals, could pass from parents to their child as a genetic disorder, but in my opinion most likely from mother to the fetus through the placenta during pregnancy. Genetics is a DNA fingerprint and has absolutely nothing to do with any type of disease except the physical structure of the human body; you cannot find disease in the DNA fingerprint.

Transfer of some carcinogens from the mother to the child will reduce in the mother the concentration of carcinogens below critical, therefore the mother will profit, development of disease in her body will be delayed and start again when all losses are replaced, which could take many years depending on the amount transferred to the fetus.

Disease will be developed only when accumulated carcinogens again reach the critical concentration. If a mother decides to have many children and shares her accumulated carcinogens with every child born from her, she might never reach the critical concentration of accumulated carcinogens and never develop the disease in her life.

The unfortunate child born from this mother will develop the disease sooner than the normal time needed for the carcinogens to reach a critical concentration for adults as some of the carcinogens were already acquired from the mother at the time of birth. Therefore, because of his or her small body size, the child needs less time to reach the critical concentration of carcinogens and start to develop the disease. This is the main reason for many youngsters getting cancer in their early years. There are many cases supporting this as when the mother, not the father, had cancer, lupus or arthritis, and the child born from this mother, had a greater chance of carrying these diseases first in latent form then activated when critical concentration was reached.

Promoter

Promoter (a piece of a destroyed cell): The initiator (carcinogen) alone cannot develop the disease. It can only prepare the body to be in readiness until agent number two, the promoter, comes along to start the development of the disease. Otherwise, the initiator will stay dormant forever.

In the development of disease, each type of initiator (carcinogen) causes one type of disease only; cancer, lupus, arthritis, asthma, etc.

But the promoter is the same for all developing diseases regardless of what type of initiator is present. Fragments of destroyed cells are promoters of disease. Promoters are produced in the body naturally during emotional situations like experiencing a tragedy, being under stress, feeling fear or hopelessness and worrying, etc. Artificial sources of the production of promoters could come from the destruction of body cells by x-rays, radioactive materials, radon gas or chemicals like the ones used in chemotherapy to destroy cancerous cells which could also destroy healthy cells. In other words, any situation or things including microorganisms and viruses capable of destroying a body cell to its fragment can be classified as a disease promoter, which can, in turn, stimulate the initiator to start to develop a disease.

Initially, initiators are in the bloodstream and circulating all over the body. The area of the body in which cancer develops depends on where the promotor was produced. Cigarette smoking cannot cause cancer; it can only produce a promoter, which causes cancer to start in the lung.

Symptoms

Almost every disease has symptoms expressed in different ways such as high temperature, cold feeling, sweating, sneezing, coughing, pale color, yellow color, discolored urine, vomiting, diarrhea, abdominal pain, arthritis pain, allergy, skin eczema, headache, back pain, dizziness and so on. There is no symptom of cancer.

For any disease to produce a symptom, a body cell must be broken, and the contents of the cell must pour into the bloodstream, which gives us a symptom. With cancer, the cell does not break open, and its contents do not pour out of the cell; therefore there is no symptom. That is the reason when cancer is discovered; it is often too late to cure it.

A cancer cell is a healthy cell connected on the surface to a promoter, and that is why the cell itself is not broken or damaged; therefore the contents of the cell does not pour into the bloodstream to give us a symptom.

Heart Cancer

Almost every organ in the body can be cancerous, such as; brain, lungs, liver, kidneys, pancreas, stomach, intestine, colon, ovaries, uterus, cervical, vaginal, prostate, testicles and so on. There is no cancer of the heart. To turn a cell of the heart cancerous, we would have to take out an electron from the cell of the heart. However, because of electromagnetic activity in the heart, it is impossible to move an electron out of the heart. Electromagnetism activity does not permit an electron to leave the atom; it keeps it in its original location; therefore, no active center is created on the surface of the cell. As a consequence, a promoter cannot be chemically connected to the surface and the cell cannot become cancerous.

The Body's Defense System

The primary function of the white blood cells is to provide a mobile system of protection for the body. All white blood cells are more or less capable of amoeboid movement. This property is especially developed in the Europhile group of the granulocytes and the monocytes. Their amoeboid capability enables them to pass through the walls of the capillaries and into the tissue spaces.

In normal blood conditions granulocytes and monocytes (types of white blood cells) move at random, but when an infective condition is created their course is directed toward that area by chemotaxis. On arriving there, they cease to move and begin a phagocytosis (a process by which phagocytes or white blood cells engulf the infection causing foreign substance or antigen) and signal for antibody production, then engulf the antigen antibody complex. Foreign substances or antigens could be inert (asbestos, broken tissue) or living microorganisms (bacteria or viruses).

If some particles are foreign for one body, that does not necessarily mean they are foreign for every human body; they could be foreign for one and self for another and vice versa (like blood groups). However, even if a macromolecule is not a normal constituent of the body, it will not act as an antigen and invoke antibody response unless it is recognized by the body as being a foreign macromolecule. The ability of the body to recognize a foreign macromolecule is not acquired until about the time of birth. Before this time the body accepts all macromolecules as its own and remembers them as its own and does not form antibodies against them.

Under favorable conditions, phagocytes are defined as the property of granulocytes and monocytes and digest inert particles and living or dead microorganisms. The three phases in phagocytes are as follows:

1. An adhesion phase, during which the phagocyte cell comes in contact with the foreign particle.

2. An ingestion phase, during which the particle is engulfed and absorbed into the cytoplasm.

3. The third phase, which features alternate possibilities that depend on the functional state of the cell and the nature of the ingested material, such as:

    A. Digestion: Ingested particle is digested (broken tissue or dead microorganism).

    B. Persistence: Foreign particles persist (asbestos, carbon dust, food preservatives, other chemicals).

    C. Multiplication: Ingested living microorganisms may proliferate inside the cytoplasm multiplying themselves and destroying the white cells (living microorganisms, HIV).

Because of their enzymes, white blood cells can degrade proteins and polysaccharides. Protein degradation is variable and relates to the type of foreign particles, type of white cells and physical conditions. This variability may explain why one antigen is destroyed by certain white cells but not by others.

In consequence, persisting foreign particles are initially in the bloodstream and circulating all over the body. They are not attacked by the defensive white blood cells unless they chemically react with normal body cells or produce altered body cells spontaneously or under the ionizing effect of radiation. This type of altered body cell is a constant target to be attacked by defensive white blood cells, engulfed, and digested, but the originating chemicals are released into the bloodstream to start the cycle all over again.

Enzyme catalyzed breakdown of the body's normal cells produces normal waste byproducts but the enzyme catalyzed breakdown of the altered cells produce foreign waste by-products. These foreign waste by-products are not large enough to be engulfed again by the white blood cells or are not broken down enough to be filtered by the kidneys, so they will stay and be stored in the body.

Seeping through tissues, the lymph bathes cells with dissolved food and oxygen molecules and eventually rejoins the bloodstream through a network of lymphatic channels. Passing through infected tissue, the lymph picks up all kinds of foreign particles, including infected and destroyed white cells transporting and depositing them in various organs such as the lymph nodes, liver or spleen and they may remain there in recognizable form for weeks. During its passage through the nodes, foreign particles are removed by the phagocyte cells. During an infection, the white blood cells greatly increase in numbers. They migrate to the sites of injury. Lymph nodes, therefore, furnish an important barrier against the spread of bacteria throughout the body and white blood cells are the defense mechanism against local infection. Immobility and fatty construction of the body will greatly interfere with the free circulation of the lymph and create additional difficulty in fighting against disease.

During an infection the great multiplication of white blood cells in a node causes the node to become enlarged and tender. When the nodes, loaded with bacteria and their byproducts, are unable any longer to cope with the situation and breakdown, the infection spreads all over the body.

A low level of foreign particles is not harmful, like in the case of urine, but might be lethal if they were allowed to accumulate in the tissues. These foreign particles and their waste by-products, mainly dissolved in the lymph, will accumulate over the years until they reach a certain critical concentration. They will then start influencing the outcome of the production of body cells.

These foreign particles once "dormant" could be very active under ionizing radiation by x-ray or radioactive materials and act as an initiator, furnishing material to start and build an altered cell. The reaction itself is catalytic and not programmed or controlled by any enzyme; therefore the products are different every time. Moreover, there is no way to control or stop them.

Depending upon the nature of the foreign particles and the location in the body where the reaction begins, they could lead to different types of illnesses like arthritis, lupus, leukemia, cancer, colitis, etc.

Any attempt to cure the disease using drugs or medicines will increase the quantity of the foreign particles and, although there may be a temporary delay, will create more complications, trouble and side effects and never cure the disease.

The only way to stop the undesirable body cell destruction or altered cell production is to reduce the concentration of the foreign particles in the body to reverse the trend of reaction. This could be achieved by using the bio-therapeutic method called Neutral Infection Absorption (NIA) to drain away all the disease-causing foreign particles from the infected body.

Metastasis

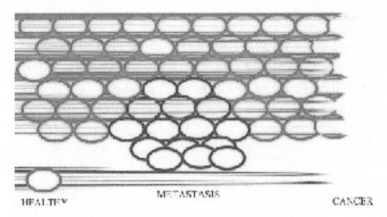

HEALTHY   METASTASIS   CANCER

Figure 4. Metastasis of Cancerous Cells

Once a healthy cell is turned into a cancerous cell it cannot stay in its pre-existing location for two reasons. Reason #1: A cancer cell is created by an initiator causing a promoter (a piece of a destroyed cell) to attach to a healthy cell. Once it is attached, the size of the now cancerous cell is increased, therefore it cannot physically stay at the same location. Reason #2: The cancerous cell is not the same as a healthy cell and therefore is seen as foreign to the surrounding healthy cells and will be rejected. Because promoters are different sizes, cancerous cells are also different sizes, and they cannot stick together; they stay loose. Cancerous cells can use the bloodstream or the lymphatic system to move around in the body. (See Figure 4.)

If the bloodstream is used for the cancerous cells to move around in the body, they will end up in the capillaries of the lungs, a very common site of cancer metastasis. If the lungs cannot contain all of the cancer cells, the overflow of cancer cells will end up in the brain.

If the lymphatic system is used, the cancer cells, traveling throughout the body, will first end up in the lymph nodes. If the lymph nodes cannot contain all of the cancer cells, the overflow of cancer cells will end up in the liver. Cancer cells trapped in the lymph nodes will be destroyed slowly. If the liver cannot contain the overflow of cancer cells, the cancer cells will move to the bones. The brain and the bones are the last stop for metastasizing (spreading) cancer cells.

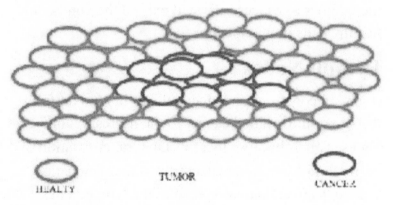

HEALTY   TUMOR   CANCER

Figure 5. Cancerous Tumor

Newly developed cancer cells will form a soft tumor. (See Figure 5.) They are like fish in a net and grow if they cannot find a way to join the circulating bloodstream or lymphatic system. In a tumor, cancer cells are loose because each of them is different since each of them has attached to a different size promoter (a piece of a destroyed cell). Different size cancer cells cannot stick together. Cancer cells in a tumor will also metastasize if the tumor cannot hold them in the sac and it bursts.

The number of cancer cells in a tumor will be more than existing healthy cells because for every healthy cell that is turned into cancer there will be the same number replaced with a new cell by dividing one of the healthy cells that surround the missing one to replace the vacated space, and this new cell can also be turned into cancer, and again another cell will be divided to replace the newly vacated space and so on. This way the number of cancer cells will exceed the number of healthy cells in that location.

Lymph Nodes

It is very common for cancer cells to first travel from the site of the original cancer to the nearest lymph nodes. This is because there is a natural circulation of tissue fluid from the organs through the lymphatic system. Cancer that has spread to the lymph nodes may cause them to swell up. It is easy to see those by self-examination if they are near the surface of the body. The swollen lymph nodes can block the circulation of tissue fluid. This can cause fluid retention and swelling in the part of the body affected. For example, swollen lymph nodes in the armpit or groin can cause swelling in the arm or leg.

Cancerous cells trapped in the lymph nodes will be slowly destroyed. If a lymph node cannot contain all of the cancer cells, the remaining cancer cells will further spread and end up in the liver or lungs. If the liver and lungs cannot contain all the cancer cells, then the remaining cancer cells will spread further and will end up in the bones and brain, the last stop for spreading cancer cells.

Autoacceleration

New cancerous cells will have different sizes and shapes and therefore will not fit in the same place. Also, the surrounding cells will see the new cancerous cells as foreign and will reject them. If cancerous cells can find a way, they will join the bloodstream or lymphatic system and circulate all over the body to create secondary sources of cancer by metastasis, or they will form a sac, like fish in a net, in the same area and grow to form a malignant tumor. The uncontrolled division of cancer cells can happen in two ways; auto acceleration and continuous division of free cancer cells.

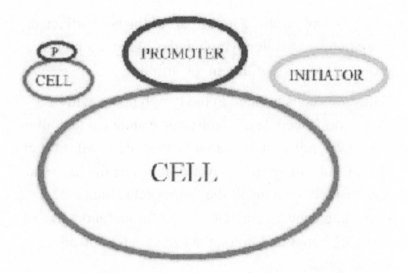

Figure 6. Autoacceleration

1. Auto acceleration happens when an initiator (carcinogen) chemically helps connect a promoter (a piece of a destroyed cell) to a healthy body cell, which turns the healthy cell into a cancerous cell. The newly created cancer cell then itself becomes an initiator increasing the number of carcinogens that already exist in the body, which turns the reaction into auto acceleration or autocatalytic. As a consequence cancer production increases. This reaction is called auto acceleration because every time a cancer cell is produced the number of initiators increases and, therefore accelerates the production of cancer cells.

The auto accelerated reaction is the main reason for the fast production of cancerous cells in the body. By the mechanism of the auto accelerated chemical reaction, a lot of healthy cells are turned into cancerous cells, which, when the cancerous cells are in a vital organ, destroys the vital organ's ability to sustain life, and, as a consequence, is the leading cause of death. Death is caused not because of too many cancerous cells but because of too few healthy cells left to sustain the function of the vital organs.

2. The other possibility of the uncontrolled division of cancer cells is when a healthy cell becomes cancerous and leaves the location and becomes a free floating cancerous cell in the lymphatic system. A cell's intent is to divide if it feels space around it and will stop dividing if there is no space. When a normal cell divides, in general, it produces two identical normal cells. However, when a cancer cell divides, two non-identical cancer cells are produced. This is because when a cancer cell divides it must, at the same time, divide the promoter and the promoter cannot be divided into two identical pieces. Therefore cancer cells are not identical, and as a consequence, they cannot stick together.

If there are many empty spaces around it, a cell will divide as many times as needed to fill all the space and will stop dividing when there is no more space. Since a cancerous cell is free and, if it is in the lymphatic system, it will circulate throughout the body by metastasis until it settles in the liver, lungs, brain or bones. Since metastasized cancerous cells rest on the surface of the lung, for instance, only one side is occupied. All the other five sides are empty, and the mechanism of cell division gets into action and starts to divide to fill all the space around it. Since a divided cancer cell creates two non-identical cancer cells that do not stick to each other, they never create a barrier around themselves to stop the division. These cancerous cells, no matter where they metastasize to, are the same as their source (original cancer). This is called uncontrollable cancer cell division by Oncologist Researchers.

A carcinogen is not a living microorganism to be killed to cure the disease; therefore we cannot use drugs to kill carcinogens or eliminate them. The only way to cure cancer is to physically remove the carcinogens out of the body by using the Neutral Infection Absorption (NIA) method. There is no alternative method to cure cancer. The NIA method is the perfect method and the only one. Because no medications are used, there are no dangerous side effects and no recurrences, which are imminent when using radiation and chemotherapy.

Breast Cancer

If a woman has enough carcinogens in her body, she will have breast cancer if she produces a promoter (a piece of a destroyed cell). If she has a condition to produce a promoter, cancer will be in the breast because in women the breast is the most sensitive organ. Removing the breast for prophylactic purposes will not stop her from having cancer, cancer will just start somewhere else. If cancerous cells can move freely they will join the lymphatic system and end up first in the nearest lymph nodes, in the armpit. If there are too many cancer cells, the remaining cells will end up in the lungs or the liver. If they cannot find a way to join the bloodstream or the lymphatic system they will develop a soft malignant tumor, like fish in a net. The first signs of cancer will be swollen lymph nodes in the armpit. Swollen lymph nodes in the armpit can cause swelling in the arm on the same side of the body.

It is not necessary to find out where the cancer is in the breast, how big the tumor is or if it has spread all over the body. We do not need to know to which part of the body cancer has spread. We only need to know if there are traces of cancer. That's enough to start the NIA treatment method immediately. Never have a mastectomy. That is not a solution, it can only delay cancer for a couple of months or years, because removing the breast will remove the carcinogens that

31

exist in the breast only, not from the bloodstream. When we start the cancer treatment with the NIA method, first all metastatic cancers (metastatic cancers have spread from where they started to other parts of the body) and carcinogens in the blood will be cleaned up, then it will stop a tumor from growing. White defensive blood cells will destroy the cancer cells slowly in the tumor.

Female Reproductive Organ's Cancer

The cause of the female reproductive organ's cancer is very clear. The first condition is to have carcinogens in the body at a critical concentration. That happens when carcinogens accumulate and reach their critical concentration in the body during many years of eating the contaminated food we consume. Once the carcinogens are at a critical concentration cancer starts when a promoter is produced in the area of the female reproduction organs. The main cause of cancer in the female reproductive organs is sperm contaminated with the Human Papilloma Virus (HPV), a sexually transmitted disease (STD), which produces a promoter. Carcinogens use the promoter to turn healthy cells into cancerous cells. All this happens during intercourse.

HPV and Vulval Cancer

Vulva cancer happens when sperm, contaminated with HPV, contaminates the entrance of the vagina. HPV contaminated sperm produces the promoter, and carcinogens use it to cause vulva cancer. [4]

HPV and Vaginal Cancer

During intercourse, if the penis is in the middle of the vagina and sperm contaminated with HPV pours into the middle of the vagina, the contaminated sperm produces the promoter, and carcinogens use it to produce vaginal cancer. [3]

HPV and Cervical Cancer

During intercourse, if the penis is in front of the cervix, but not touching it, and sperm contaminated with HPV pours onto the cervix, the contaminated sperm produces the promoter, and carcinogens use it to produce cervical cancer. [2]

HPV and Uterus Cancer

During intercourse, if the penis is in deep, firmly touching the cervix, and sperm contaminated with HPV pours into the uterus with low pressure, the contaminated sperm produces the promoter, and carcinogens use it to produce uterine cancer.

HPV and Ovarian Cancer

During intercourse, if the penis is in deep, firmly touching the cervix, and sperm contaminated with HPV pours into the uterus with high pressure and reaches the fallopian tubes, the contaminated sperm produces the promoter, and carcinogens use it to produce ovarian cancer.

HPV and Anal Cancer

During anal intercourse when sperm, contaminated with HPV, contaminates the anus it creates anal cancer. HPV contaminated sperm produces the promoter, and carcinogens use it to cause anal cancer. [5]

Lung Cancer

Cigarette smoking never caused and never will cause cancer. It can only produce a promoter (a piece of a destroyed cell). If a person has enough carcinogens in their body, then cigarette smoking will help to start cancer in the lungs. If a person chews tobacco, the tobacco will help to start cancer in the mouth because tobacco produces a promoter. If cancer metastasized from another primary source of cancer, then a non-smoker will have secondary cancer in the lungs. Both smokers and non-smokers are subject to having lung cancer from a lung infection like the flu or tuberculosis. The lungs are the most vulnerable organs for metastasizing (spreading) cancer. This is because the blood from most parts of the body flows back to the heart and then to the lungs before it goes to any other organ. Cancer cells that have found their way into the bloodstream can get stuck in the tiny capillaries of the lungs. Whether the cancer is primary for smokers or secondary for non-smokers, if the cancer source establishes itself in the lungs it usually contains water and physicians can drain the fluid by putting in a needle or a thin tube. Unless you are using the NIA method to stop the fluid from collecting, it will build up again and again. When cancer establishes itself in the lungs, there is a very good possibility of getting an infection so that treatment will start with an antibiotic.

Recently there has been too much talk about cigarette smoking causing lung cancer. It is a baseless lie. Cigarette smoking does not cause cancer. It can only produce promoters, which help to cause cancer if carcinogens exist in the body at a critical concentration. My father started to smoke cigarettes when he was 12 years old. His father, my grandfather, was a tobacco merchant, so cigarettes were readily available. My father smoked cigarettes 12 hours a day and never had any problem with his lungs. He died of natural causes at 80 years old. If cigarette smoking causes lung cancer the 40 to 50 million Americans who are smoking cigarettes should die of lung cancer. In reality, only 400 thousand a year die from lung cancer.

You cannot blame only cigarette smoking for it since there are many other reasons. Such as metastasis from original sites of other types of cancer.

I do not mean to encourage smoking. I do not smoke, and I do not like smokers. It is not a good habit, but nobody can deny scientific results, and nobody has the right to falsify facts to deny smoking. Women are the flowers of our life; smokers are the weeds.

Stomach Cancer

Helicobacter Pylori Infection and Cancer

Helicobacter Pylori (H. pylori) is a spiral bacterium that specifically and selectively resides beneath the mucous layer next to the stomach and duodenum. The bacterium invades the stomach lining causing chronic gastritis. H. pylori produce promoters; therefore it causes most stomach cancers. Metastasis from pancreatic cancer can cause stomach cancer also.

H. pylori infection usually causes pain at night when the stomach is empty, and the H. pylori start to irritate the wall of the stomach. There is some relief of pain when food is consumed and a recurrence of the pain in two to four hours when the stomach is empty again. The irritation produces promoters, which are used by carcinogens to turn healthy cells into cancerous cells.

There are highly effective treatments for the H. pylori infection, and evidence from trials suggests a reduction in gastric cancer risk with the eradication of H. pylori. Eradication of H. pylori generally requires a combination of antibiotics and an acid-blocker/proton pump inhibitor. Current medical regimens should achieve a greater than 85 percent eradication of H. pylori infection after one to two weeks of treatment.

With the eradication of H. pylori, the production of the promoters stops, and the carcinogens stop turning healthy cells into cancerous cells because of insufficient promoters. By using the NIA method, you will eliminate carcinogens and cancer will never come back again even if H. pylori is still there because the cancer was caused by carcinogens, not by H. pylori bacterium. [6]

Liver Cancer

Many cancers spread to the liver. The cancers of the digestive system are most likely to spread to the liver because the lymph from the digestive system circulates through the capillaries of the liver before it goes back to the heart and then to the lungs. So it is common for digestive system cancers that have spread to the liver to cause liver cancer.

In fact, the liver is the second most common site of cancer metastasis after the lungs.

There are many ways cancer in the liver can cause ascites (abnormal accumulation of fluid). Cancer may be blocking the normal lymph flow through the liver causing a back pressure of the fluid. The healthy liver makes proteins that circulate in the blood. The proteins help to keep the fluid in the bloodstream and stop it from leaking out into the tissues. If the liver is damaged, it may not be making enough of these proteins, and so fluid tends to leak out and collect in the abdomen or other parts of the body, such as the feet and ankles. Excess fluid can be drained from inside the abdomen by putting in a needle. But unless they can stop the fluid from collecting, it will build up again and again. Only the NIA method can fix the problem.

Bone Cancer

Bone cancer cannot be the primary source of cancer, but some cancers quite often spread to the bones. The most common secondary cancer in the bones of the lower part of the body is from prostate cancer, testicular cancer, cervical and uterus cancers. Secondary cancer in the bones of the upper part of the body come from breast cancer and lung cancer.

Pancreatic Cancer

Sometimes it is very difficult to guess where cancer will start, but one thing we can say is that cancer will start where ever in the body promoters are being produced. From my own experience, when I had pancreatic cancer, metastasis occurred in my stomach, intestine and the duct connecting the pancreas to the stomach, and, of course, it could have ended up in the liver also. Read the story about my own pancreatic cancer below.

My Experience With Pancreatic Cancer

I was treating people who had various incurable diseases, starting with Rheumatoid Arthritis, Rheumatism, Breast cancer and so on, but I had never experienced any incurable disease myself and had been dreaming of having a first-hand experience. All the people who used my NIA method previously were others who told me their doctor said they had breast cancer that had spread all over their body and after the NIA treatment, their doctor said they didn't have cancer, but I could not prove it on myself.

Then, on September 23, 2003, I had pain in my upper abdomen. The next day I started vomiting and had diarrhea. My color was yellow, and my urine was as black as coffee. My physician admitted me to St. Luke's Roosevelt Hospital in Manhattan, NY. All the medication to stop the vomiting and diarrhea failed to help. I could not eat anything and was running to the toilet 6-7 times a day. I lost 53 pounds in seven days — I went from weighing 195 pounds to 142 pounds.

Nobody could find out what the problem was; what was going on.

Finally, on September 29, 2003, my doctors decided to perform surgery to correct my problems. During surgery, the doctors found that I had pancreatic cancer. After five and a half hours of surgery, they removed both ends of my pancreas, removed a tumor that was blocking the duct between my pancreas and stomach, removed a third of my cancerous stomach and removed my gall bladder that contained stones. In the end, the five participant doctors recommended that my wife prepare a funeral for me, just in case. My wife told me that we do not have enough cash in the bank for a funeral. I said, "It is very simple, we do not have money for a funeral, so I will not die, so we will not need money for a funeral."

After I woke up from the surgery my main surgeon, Dr. Fadi F. Attiyeh, M.D., told me I had pancreatic cancer. I told him very nicely that I was happy. He said he was very serious and said chemotherapy was the only hope to save my life. I rejected it immediately and asked him to discharge me from the hospital so that I could go home. At home, I immediately started my NIA treatment, and after two months my blood test to find traces of cancer was negative and is still negative. In the UK only five percent of people with my kind of pancreatic cancer survive, and in the US only four percent survive.

Brain Cancer

Brain cancer is most possibly caused by metastasis from lung cancer. The most common symptoms of cancer that spread to the brain are; headaches and feeling sick. These symptoms are caused because the growing cancer tumor in the brain is taking up space.

The space for the brain is limited by the skull, so the growing cancer tumor causes an increase in pressure inside the skull. This is called raised intracranial pressure.

Male Reproductive Organ's Cancer

Testicular Cancer

Testicular cancer usually starts by the Human Papilloma Virus (HPV), a sexually transmitted disease (STD), which can produce a promoter in the testicle. If there are enough carcinogens at a critical concentration in the body cancer is inevitable. Testicular cancer often spreads to the nearest lymph nodes in the groin from primary cancer. Then, from there to the bones. Sperm produced in testicles infected with HPV will contain HPV and will cause HPV to spread to female partners during intercourse if sexual activity is not protected.

Prostate Cancer

If a man has enough carcinogens in his body, then he will have prostate cancer if he produces a promoter. If he has the condition to produce a promoter, it will be in the prostate because for a man the prostate is the most sensitive organ. If cancerous cells can move freely they will join the circulating lymphatic system and then, on their way, be trapped in the lymph nodes of the groin. Swollen lymph nodes can block the circulation of tissue fluid. Swollen lymph nodes in the groin can cause swelling in the leg. If the accumulated sperm in the prostate is infected with HPV of the testicle, then cancer will be prostate cancer. In some cases, prostate cancer spreads to the bone unexpectedly.

HPV and Penile Cancer

During intercourse, if the vagina is infected with HPV then the penis is washed with HPV and will produce a promoter on the penis and cause penile cancer when a critical concentration of carcinogens or more are in the body.

Almost 90% of in situ and 70% of invasive penile tumor samples are positive for HPV DNA. Men with antibodies to HPV16 have double the risk of invasive penile cancer compared with men without antibodies. [1]

Circumcision

The following is my personal opinion to explain the reason, benefit and the need for circumcision, why it happened and where it started. I was born in the Middle East, and from my own experience, I know that on hot summer days sperm production is at its peak and the prostate is full and overflowing. If the sperm is not used on time because a man is not married or not visiting a prostitute or relieving the prostate by other means, sperm tends to leak, and this leak accumulates at the tip of the penis under the foreskin. If this leakage is not washed or wiped up on time, the penis will get infected.

Thousands of years ago in the Middle East and North Africa hygiene was very poor, and there was a lack of water and soap. At that time smart people figured out a solution to avoid infection of the penis. They introduced circumcision as the best solution, particularly in the hot countries of the Middle East and North Africa, where circumcision became not only routine but the main identity for Muslims and Jews. During WW2 Hitler used circumcision to identify Jews from Christians.

Now we have just entered the 21st Century, and conditions have changed dramatically all over the world, particularly in the Middle East and North Africa, so we no longer need circumcision. When it was first introduced circumcision not only became a routine practice it also became part of the religion for Muslims and Jews. At that time in history the only way to enforce a solution for better health was through religion so the process of circumcision became a religious ceremony. Then circumcision became a political tool also, as many hospitals in the U.S. forcibly practiced circumcision as a tool to fool and confuse the next "Hitler" from identifying Jews from Christians.

We do not need circumcision anymore. It has no benefit and, in some circumstances, may infect the woman. The foreskin keeps the tip of the penis covered, lubricated, sensitive and clean. Circumcised penis' lose their sensitivity, are not covered and protected, are not lubricated, and the absence of it could irritate and introduce infection to the vagina during intercourse. Both male and female circumcision is not acceptable and must be stopped.

Rheumatoid Arthritis

If we compare Rheumatoid Arthritis to other diseases, we find that it has a mechanism similar to cancer. The only difference is the carcinogen. This time the carcinogen attacks only the cartilage of the joints turning cells of cartilage into cancerous cells which get loose and spread all over the body by metastasis, thinning the cartilage or tearing it down completely.

If healthy cartilage cells turn cancerous, but can not get loose or get loose but can not join the bloodstream, they will form a soft malignant tumor around the joints and the defensive white cells will attack them in this area causing it to swell and to have redness around the joints, which is common for Rheumatoid Arthritis.

Altered cells of cartilage are not a part of a life-sustaining organ. Therefore they do not cause death because they are attacking only cartilage, which is not an important life-sustaining functional organ. A 100% cure is available if you use the "Neutral Infection Absorption" method.

HIV and Cancer

Human Immunodeficiency Virus (HIV), like other infections, can only produce a promoter. It is likely that the weakened immune system of someone with AIDS allows and helps the growth of a tumor quickly. HIV/AIDS cannot cause cancer if there are not carcinogens in the body at a critical concentration. The NIA method is the best method to cure HIV/AIDS disease. [7]

Comparison

There are two groups of diseases. One caused by viral bacteria and the other by particle chemicals.

The first group of diseases (venereal, flu, etc.) is initiated by a living microorganism like viruses and bacterium. In this group, diseases are transferable from one person to another by physical contact or by air.

The second group of diseases (cancer, arthritis, etc.) are caused by particles and chemicals (asbestos, food preservatives, etc.). These diseases are not transferable by contact or by air.

If you have a single virus in your body, you never feel the symptoms of the disease. A virus, using a cell's internal duplication mechanism, duplicates itself and accumulates in the body. You do not feel the disease, but when it reaches a certain "critical" amount of viruses, you will experience the full symptoms of the disease.

To reach the "critical" amount of viruses it could take between a few minutes to a few hours.

The same is true for a microorganism. The only difference is that a microorganism is not using a cell's duplication mechanism. Instead, it is using the cell as a nutrient and reproducing itself.

To cure these types of viral and bacterial diseases, since they are living microorganisms, we can use medicine to kill or immobilize the viruses and the bacterium in addition to the body's defense system.

In diseases caused by particles and chemicals, the mechanism is different. This time there is no duplication or reproduction. Instead, accumulation must reach the "critical" amount to cause disease, which takes years.

The kind of chemicals that cause "incurable" disease comes from inside the body and accumulates through the food we consume to survive. The Neutral Infection Absorption (NIA) method is the only method to cure these incurable diseases. There is no alternative. It is the only way to cure these diseases.

To try to cure these kinds of diseases by using radiation or chemotherapy can only cause cancer or accelerate existing cancer and never cure it because radiation and chemotherapy do not eliminate the cause of disease, which is carcinogens.

Radiation and chemotherapy kill the cancerous cells and also healthy cells and leaves the carcinogens to start all over again. Imagine if you treated a bacterial disease by destroying just the damaged cells and left the bacteria alive to start damaging more and more cells.

List of Diseases Cured Using NIA

1. Cancer Category: breast, liver, spleen, lung, pancreatic, stomach, intestinal, colon, kidney, vulvar, vaginal, cervical, uterine, ovarian, leukemia, skin, bone, brain, prostate, testicle, bladder, lymph nodes, mouth, in one word ALL cancer diseases.

2. Rheumatoid Arthritis Category: Rheumatoid Arthritis, Rheumatism, Arthritis, Emphysema, Glaucoma, Bronchitis, Asthma, Lupus, Colitis, and all Arthritic related diseases.

3. HIV/AIDS can be cured if you use the (NIA) Neutral Infection Absorption method.

NIA Treatment Method Instructions
Treatment Supplies

For the first time:

1. Shaving razor

2. Plastic ring (25 mm in diameter)

or wedding band

3. Adhesive tape

4. Fresh garlic

5. Garlic Crusher

6. Plastic Sheet (fold & stick together Scotch shipping tape to make a 2X2" plastic sheet)

7. Nail Scissors

8. Tweezers

For everyday use:

1. Alcohol

2. Cotton ball

3. Chickpeas

4. Cabbage

5. Absorbent paper sandwiches (cut from white, unscented paper towels or napkins)

6. Adhesive tape

7. Elastic bandage

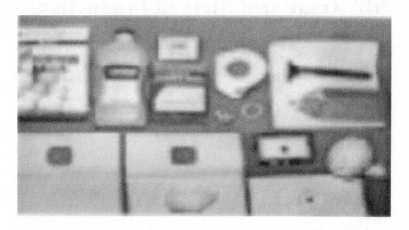

Picture 1. The material used during treatment.

Creation of A Wound for NIA Treatment

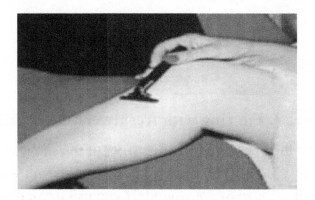

Picture 2. Shave location to start the treatment.

We have to make a wound to start the NIA treatment. First, we have to choose the location; the area has to be on soft muscle far from the bone. Calves are the most practical place to make the wound than anywhere else on the body; it's easier to take care of without help. To make it easier, if you are left handed start on your right calf and if you are right handed start on your left calf. Shave the location approximately 6 to 8 centimeters (3 inches) in diameter leaving the area of the wound to be directly in the center.

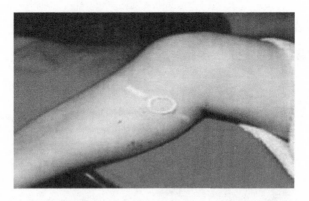

Picture 3. Fill ring with freshly crushed garlic.

Secure the plastic ring in the center of the shaved area with two pieces of adhesive tape. A plastic ring is used to limit the size of the wound. If you cannot find a plastic ring, you can use a wedding band. Fill the ring evenly with freshly crushed garlic, as high as the thickness of the ring. Cover the ring with a sheet of plastic so that the juice of the garlic will stay inside the ring and create a blister after 6 to 8 hours.

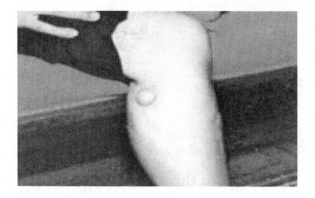

Picture 4. Blister caused by crushed garlic.

After 6 to 8 hours the blister will be ready.

To avoid infection clean up around the blister with alcohol before peeling off the skin. First, make a small cut with the nail scissors, then peel the skin off. Sometimes you don't see the blister because it formed and burst, so you have to remove the skin of the blister by scratching the area with the sharp end of the nail scissors to remove the dead skin.

Never touch or treat the inside of the wound with alcohol or peroxide. Always wash your hands before replacing the chickpeas. You do not need to wash the chickpeas or the cabbage.

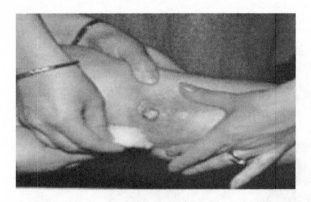

Picture 5. Chickpea is in the wound.

The wound is ready. Place a chickpea in the center of the wound and cover it with a prepared sandwich of cabbage (fresh from the refrigeration) and absorbing paper, so that the inside surface of the cabbage, the clean side, faces the wound, then bind it with an elastic bandage tight enough so it will not slip down when you walk. Note: The "sandwich" is a 5.5 X 3.5 inch folded sheet of white, unscented paper towel or napkin with a round or diamond shaped hole cut out of the middle of one side. The cabbage is placed inside the fold so the cabbage shows through the hole and faces the wound.

Since saliva destroys bacteria and will prevent an accidental infection moisten the first dry chickpea with the saliva from your mouth for a couple of seconds and then place it in the wound. This is needed because the first chickpea in the wound has not yet established a flow of lymph fluid from inside the body to the outside. This flow will not give the infection a chance to go inside the body. The moistening of the first chickpea only is needed, you do not need to repeat moistening the chickpeas every day. Only the first one.

The body will feel the presence of the foreign substance and will fight against it by sending the proper body cells to this area to neutralize it.

The chickpea will absorb the lymphatic fluid and the carcinogens and establish the flow of liquid from inside the body to the outside until it gets saturated. The chickpea keeps the wound alive and will not let it heal.

The absorbing paper in the sandwich will absorb any excess of fluid. The cabbage will keep moisture in, which will prevent the rim of the wound from becoming dry and sticky. This will facilitate the exchange of the chickpeas.

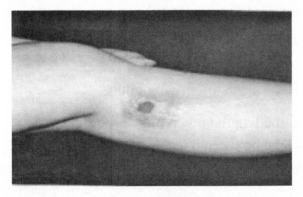

Picture 6. Wound without chickpea.

The next day, after 24 hours, open the wound and take out the saturated chickpea. Clean up around the wound with alcohol, insert another dry chickpea in the wound and cover it with a new clean sandwich of cabbage and absorbing paper. Then, over the absorbing paper, bind it with an elastic bandage. Repeat the same process again every 24 hours for two days, then begin replacing the chickpea every 12 hours.

However, if the flow of the fluid is extensive and saturation of the chickpea comes earlier, you may replace the chickpea before two days and begin the 12-hour schedule.

The sandwich of absorbing paper and cabbage has to be replaced by a new one every time the saturated chickpea is replaced. By replacing saturated chickpeas with dry ones, we are removing carcinogens and other disease-causing chemicals that have been absorbed into the chickpeas.

This procedure has to be continued again and again until the body is cleared of all impurities from foreign substances.

The blood will be clean after two months.

Depending on the length and complication of the illness it will take between 6 to 24 months to remove all the trouble causing particles and chemicals from all over the body.

When you take a shower, first take a shower then change and replace the chickpea. Do not take a shower with an open wound. The wound will get infected if you leave it open more than one minute without a chickpea, so replace the dry one immediately without delay.

The time of termination cannot be predicted. Signs that it is time to terminate the treatment: if pus and infected blood are no longer coming out of the wound, the color of the wound is normal, and (the main thing) if you feel better.

To terminate the treatment the last chickpea has to be removed, and the wound kept empty, but the replacement of the cabbage and absorbing paper must be continued for many days until the wound is healed or you may treat it as a common wound by using antibacterial ointment.

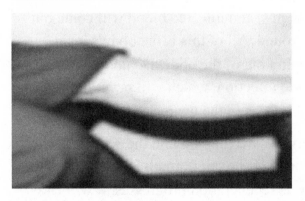

Picture 7. Closed wound after treatment.

The sole danger in this method is an outside infection gaining entrance to the wound when there is no chickpea inside the wound. With a chickpea inside the wound, the wound never gets infected, and it is safe. Certain natural infection is permissible during treatment, but you must be very careful when the wound is treated without the chickpea.

Since 1943 I have been testing this method to cure all types of so called "incurable" diseases. Most of the patients were my family members, including my mother, myself and my wife or close relatives and the diseases were arthritis related. Recuperation in all cases went up to 100%, and there has been no recurrence recorded. Since no drugs or medicines are used in this method there were no side effects as there are in medical treatments, where side effects are imminent in most cases.

You have to expect the following during treatment: a muddy liquid, pus, and infected blood will come out through the wound. All of this is the body's inside infection coming out of the body. Do not confuse these with an outside infection, which will never happen as long as a chickpea is in the wound.

Discoloration and swelling around the wound, severe pain, and a bad odor are all normal. Do not panic. All will go away as recuperation progresses. It will take time, be patient.

If the chickpea sticks in the wound, never try to pull it out by using force. If the chickpea is not saturated and will not come out easily, let the chickpea stay in the wound for another day until it gets saturated and pops out when you press around the wound with your fingers.

Before changing the chickpea, you can take a shower or swim in the sea. Then, you can change the chickpea, cabbage and paper sandwich, and the wet elastic bandage with absolutely no problem.

To terminate the treatment the last chickpea has to be removed and the wound kept empty. Continue covering the wound with the cabbage, absorbing paper sandwich, and the elastic bandage as you were doing every day. Continue this process for many days until the wound heals by itself.

If there is too much infection around the wound, healing will take a little longer until all the infection comes out completely or you may treat it as a common wound with an antibacterial medicine.

Conclusion

To cure cancer, we have to eliminate the cause. Cancer is caused by carcinogens, which were accumulated in the body during many years from the food we consumed.

Since the carcinogens are not living microorganisms, we cannot use drugs to eliminate them by killing them. We have to physically remove them from the body to eliminate the cause.

The only natural treatment method, which can remove carcinogens from the body is the Neutral Infection Absorption (NIA) method, which is the only method in the world that cures cancer. There is no alternative or substitute, and it is a perfect method and the only one.

When using the NIA method, we make an artificial wound to access inside the body, place a chickpea in the wound to keep the wound alive, establish a flow of liquid outward and absorb the carcinogens with the chickpea. We cover the chickpea with a piece of fresh cabbage to keep moisture around the wound, so it stays soft, so the replacement of the saturated chickpea with a dry one is easy and painless.

First, the presence of the chickpea in the wound keeps the wound alive and active and prevents the wound from being healed. Second, the chickpea causes the body's immune system to get into action, pushing all carcinogens, including cancerous cells and all other foreign particles, which do not belong to the body and could even do harm, toward the wound and discards them out of the body.

In two months the blood is free of carcinogens and cancerous cells, but to clean up all over the body, it will take at least six months. Then the disease will be cured 100%. In some cases, it will take a little longer, especially if the disease is many years old or has been treated with radiation and chemotherapy, but it will be cured if it is not too late or if the damage is irreversible.

During this treatment, you can see muddy liquid, pus, and infected blood coming out of the wound and it smells very bad.

If too much infection has accumulated around the wound, you will see discoloring of the skin and swelling, but it will go away as soon as the infection gets out. It happens because too much infection is coming around the wound waiting to get out and the wound is taking them out too slowly.

Sooner or later all infection will get out, and the swelling will go away. The wound itself never gets infected because the liquid flows outward.

During treatment, when pus or infected blood is coming out, it will cause you a lot of pain so you can take a painkiller for relief, but never any x-rays or medications intended to cure cancer because radiation and chemotherapy can only cause cancer or accelerate existing cancer and never cure it.

Also not recommended are home remedies, vitamins, hormonal and/or herbal treatments as they also may slow down or stop the treatment.

WARNING. In the case of diabetes take precaution when using the NIA method. Strictly control the sugar level to heal the wound successfully, and there will be no problem.

Magnetic Resonance Imaging (MRI)

Normal cells in the body are stable, balanced and have zero polarity but as soon as a healthy cell turns into a cancerous cell everything changes.

Cancerous cells are not stable, not balanced and have polarity.

This is the reason an MRI can detect cancerous cells, and only my suggested model represents them. (See Figure 7.)

When we send an impulse to normal cells, they stop, they have zero relaxation time, but cancerous cells, because of polarity and irregular shape, have a certain long relaxation time, so the MRI is detecting the differences of relaxation times between normal and cancerous cells and that gives us the locations of these cells.

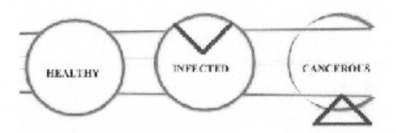

Figure 7. Magnetic Resonance Imaging (MRI)

I like to demonstrate the relaxation time of normal, damaged by bacteria (infected), and cancerous cells on a prepared model of Compact Discs. (See Figure 7.)

The healthy disc represents normal cells. They are stable and have zero polarity and zero relaxation time. When I send an impulse, the disc stops immediately.

The infected disc represents a cell damaged by bacteria, which is partially unbalanced, with very weak polarity; therefore it has close to zero relaxation time. When I send an impulse, the disc stops, but not immediately.

The cancer disc represents cancerous cells, which are polar, irregular and unstable. When I send an impulse, the disc stops only after a certain long relaxation time. These experiments show how an MRI works to detect cancerous cells.

Recommendations

At least since 1900 all the research, by Oncologists and Rheumatoid Arthritis specialists, in the fields of Cancer and Rheumatoid Arthritis, was to *not* find a cure for these diseases ensuring that the oncologists and other specialists keep their jobs and incomes forever because if they find a cure, they will have to shut down all the research centers.

Because I am a physicist and not a physician, I was not interested in continuing the research, so I found a cure for these illnesses.

The NIA method is universal. It is not a medicine for a specific illness; therefore you do not have to know specific names of the cancer illness. You do not need to know where the primary sources of the cancer are or to which part of the body it metastasized.

You do not need to have expensive tests like an MRI, CAT SCAN, PET/SCAN, X-RAYS, SONOGRAM, and others, which can only harm you more.

If you just know that you have cancer or Rheumatoid Arthritis, it is enough to start the NIA treatment, because the NIA treatment cleans up all the particles and chemicals that do not belong in the body and are causing the illness. In general, any illnesses that are incurable by medicine, the NIA method will cure 100%.

Three Reasons to Use the NIA Method

1. If you are healthy and you want to avoid Cancer and Rheumatoid Arthritis, you better use the NIA method at least for six months for prophylactic purposes because no matter what you do you will have carcinogens in your body accumulated from the food you eat.

2. If you already have the illness do absolutely nothing. Do not use any medicine to cure it. Use only the NIA method and your recuperation will be 100% without any complications, problems, or recurrence.

3. If you want a healthy baby without any medical problems: before conceiving (mother to be, not the father) must use the NIA method at least for six months to clean up the blood that will be feeding the fetus. Clean blood grows a healthy baby. If you cannot conceive, the NIA method solves the problem after six months of treatment. With the NIA method, you can have a healthy baby. Many women who had infertility successfully conceived and had a healthy baby after six months on the NIA method.

Very Important Advice for Everyone
Vaccination

Diseases can be cured, but it is more important to prevent them. To prevent diseases, scientists invented vaccinations. Each vaccination can only be used for a single virus. If you want to vaccinate for many viruses you have to make a vaccine for each virus, but sometimes the virus mutates, and the vaccine is no longer effective to prevent the disease, so you have to make a new vaccine for the mutated virus. Preparing a vaccine sometimes takes years.

In the case of chemical diseases, a vaccine cannot be used since a virus is not involved in inducing a chemical disease. A vaccine is prepared for viruses only. If you use the NIA method, which eliminates all chemical disease causing carcinogens, you will get better than a vaccine type of prevention, since the blood will be clean of all kinds of carcinogens.

After using the NIA method all cancer and rheumatoid diseases have been cured for life except cancer, which will only start again when the carcinogens get to a critical concentration, naturally, not from a previous cancer, only from new carcinogens we get from the food we consume. At the end of 10 to 15 years, if you repeat the NIA treatment again for prophylactic purposes, you prevent having cancer for another 10 to 15 years.

After using the NIA method, the following diseases are cured for life: Rheumatoid Arthritis, Rheumatism, Arthritis, Bronchitis, Asthma, and Emphysema never come back.

Also, NIA prevents Alzheimer's and Parkinson's diseases.

Please do not hesitate to use the NIA method for prophylactic purposes.

The NIA method is the best way to prevent cancer since cancer often has no symptoms and when it's discovered it could be too late (irreversible), therefore it is much wiser to use the NIA method every 10 to 15 years and be safe and healthy for life. And it is free. I am telling you, the NIA method cures "incurable" diseases 100%, but cannot bring you back from the funeral home. Therefore use it for prophylactic purposes and be safe.

You have one life to live, do not count on a second one. Ladies, please give us healthy babies. Use the NIA method for six months at least then conceive to have a trouble free healthy baby.

Regular Check-ups

A regular medical check-up is an unnecessary waste of time for both patient and physician. The time could be used for more important things such as helping already sick people who need immediate help.

No one physician can say when and what kind of illness you are going to have unless it happens. If regular check-ups could help to prevent illness from occurring, the physician himself would not get any disease and would die a natural death.

When you go for a check-up, you have to tell the doctor what kind of complaint you have; the doctor does not tell you.

Suppose during a checkup, by magic a physician found out that tomorrow you are going to have Rheumatoid Arthritis. He couldn't stop it from occurring or prevent it in any way, and if it happened, the physician has no cure for it. So what is the importance of a check-up to prevent illness from occurring?

If you have early detected breast cancer what will the oncologist do? Recommend a mastectomy, which is not a cure and the oncologist has no means to eliminate carcinogens to cure the disease, only the NIA method can do that.

No one can convince me that regular check-ups help us avoid unconfirmed illnesses and no one can provide proof that illness would not occur if they had regular check-ups.

There are thousands of cases where patients were rated 100% healthy by family doctors who later had a heart attack and died, or had other "incurable" diseases for which physicians have neither explanation nor cure.

The best thing is to be healthy and prevent many diseases from occurring by just keeping calm so as not to produce promoters so carcinogens, which you always have in your body, cannot use them to turn healthy cells into cancerous ones.

The use of the NIA method, for prophylactic purposes, is the best and only way to avoid all the "incurable" diseases from occurring and keep your health in the best disease-proof shape, except for inevitable, natural viral infections against which the body's defense system will take prompt action.

Lifestyle and Cancer Risk

In the medical literature, you read all kinds of baseless talk about different lifestyles to prevent and cure cancer. Not one of them has any proof that their claims are true. My mechanism of the development of cancer shows that prevention and the cure for cancer solely involves a method to eliminate carcinogens from the body; it is Neutral Infection Absorption (NIA) method. There is no substitute or alternative. There is no lifestyle that can eliminate carcinogens to prevent or cure cancer.

Examples of lifestyles that supposedly cause cancer include: using tobacco, excess body weight, lack of physical activity, hormones, too much sunlight, occupations, infections and the standard American diet (SAD).

Diet has nothing to do with preventing or curing cancer. Consuming selective foods cannot prevent nor cure cancer. The main problem is not the food; it is what kind of chemicals exist in the food, like in fruits and vegetables or processed food preservatives.

Some people claim you have to consume organic food to be healthy. Please do not fool yourself. There is no organic food anymore. All the claims are a dirty business to fool people to make money. One organic food is the organic tomato, which looks healthy and never gets spoiled. That is correct because it is so tasteless and void of nutrition that the worm refuses to eat it. Worms like only the best and tastiest tomatoes and that is the reason the best tomatoes get spoiled. You are better off consuming the cheapest food and then eliminating the carcinogens and chemicals you have consumed with the fruits and vegetables by using the NIA method.

Nutrition

Which food is good or bad, has high nutrition or low? You do not need to take it to a laboratory to test it to find out. We have the ideal, most super perfect laboratory right in our body — our mouth, which gives us instant test results and forces us to reject it if it is bad for our stomach or eat it if it will not harm us.

Just look at the face of a baby. If you give the baby some nutrition, their tongue instantly tells the baby whether to eat it or reject it. You can see on the face of the baby: eat it if it's good, reject it if it's not. If it's not, they will not accept it for their digestion.

If a baby decides to eat a bad food the result will be vomiting, so do not force a baby to eat when its mouth laboratory says "no." That means at this point that particular food is not acceptable because of some problem with their stomach, but try later, many times, until their stomach accepts that food.

Anyway, this problem does not mean that the food is bad. No, it's that the food is bad at that moment only because of a stomach problem. Later, that problem will be corrected, and the food will be accepted.

Our tongue tells us immediately which food is good or bad. Try a regular strawberry and a genetically modified (GM) strawberry. The regular strawberry smells fantastic and tastes very good. Then try a GM strawberry. It does not smell at all and tastes like eating plastic.

The conclusion is that normal food has a high nutrition content and we enjoy eating it, and GM food has less nutrition, will not harm you, and you will not enjoy eating it. Nature created only the best food. Any change by man will only change it for the worst. Nobody can create better food than nature.

We have another good sign to tell us which foods are good for us. For instance, a regular tomato smells good, has a high nutrition content and tastes good. The GM tomato looks good but tastes bad and contains fewer nutrients. You can fool people into eating the GM tomato, but you cannot fool worms. Worms eat only the best, and that's the reason a good tomato gets damaged, disfigured, or "spoiled" — worms eat them — and worms refuse to eat GM tomatoes because GM tomatoes have been "genetically modified" to not appeal to worms.

I experienced stomach problems myself. When the stomach has a problem and cannot digest a food, it will reject it from the beginning. When there is a problem, the tongue will not accept the food, but later when the stomach problem is fixed, the tongue will accept the same food that was rejected before.

Once I ate a beef lung shish kebab (barbecue) and caught a cold. At that time I had a stomach problem and anytime after that when I saw lung kebabs I wanted to vomit, but I still wanted to eat them. The next time I tried to eat them when I put the lung kebab to my mouth I wanted to vomit. I tried again weeks later. I put the lung kebab in my mouth and chewed. As soon as I wanted to swallow, I vomited. Later I tried again. This time I could swallow with no problem as my stomach accepted it because my stomach problem had fixed itself without any remedy. You can try again and again, and in the end, the stomach will be fixed and accept the food.

In 2003 I had pancreatic cancer, For seven consecutive days I was vomiting and had diarrhea. In seven days I lost 53 pounds. One-third of my cancerous stomach was removed. Anything I tried to eat caused vomiting. I tried many foods, and I could not eat any of them. Then I asked my wife to give me some mortadella, which was my most favorite food. When I put it in my mouth, I felt as though I was eating poison. So that I also could not eat. Finally, I tried yogurt, and it was perfect. So I ate yogurt for one month until my stomach was fixed and accepting regular food again.

On Thanksgiving Day my niece prepared a turkey. I picked up one big leg and started to eat. Everybody was looking at me, expecting me to have to vomit. I was so hungry I ate the whole leg without any problem. Being contrary I looked for another piece of turkey to eat, but the people around me did not permit it. This experience also shows that if your stomach has a problem, it will not accept certain foods, but later when the problem has been fixed by itself, it begins to accept those foods again.

I never listen to doctors about what food to eat or not eat. I listen to my stomach. Sometimes my stomach tells me I need salt and I add extra salt to my food. After a while, my stomach tells me I've had enough, and I feel salt tastes unpleasant and I stop using extra salt and go back to my normal usage. Then, weeks later, my stomach tells me I need sweets, so I obey my stomach and start to eat all kinds of jams and sweets, add double the amount of sugar to my tea and coffee, add sugar to milk to drink. Then slowly I feel sweets are bothering me and I stop using the extra amount and go back to using my normal amount.

Listen to your stomach. That is the best way to keep your body healthy. If you feel thirsty drink water or juice if you feel hot eat ice cream, do not listen to other people's food recommendations, fulfill your stomach's recommendations to keep your health. Amen.

Survey of Unorthodox Cancer Treatments

Everyone has their own idea of what it means to be a "quack." To most of us, it means someone who peddles useless products at exorbitant prices.

In recent years the term has been widened to include anyone who promotes a treatment which is not in complete accord with the policies or attitudes of organized medicine.

People who are against fluoridation, no matter what their background, are classified by some as quacks; those who are convinced of the power of vitamin E are called quacks; an advocate of natural food in the diet is labeled a quack, etc.

But the term, in its most damning sense, is reserved for those who would presume to treat cancer using anything but surgery, radiation and/or chemotherapy.

It might be an untrained country boy who has treated his local neighbors with a homemade remedy, or a bona tide researcher who has tested his treatment in a hundred scientific ways.

If the medical fraternity frowns on the treatment, the treatment is finished. The developer and his associates are branded as quacks. Your doctor will be told it is a worthless treatment. He might run into serious professional trouble if he uses it.

Actually, how good is the treatment? Medical authorities say it is no good. The researcher says it is beneficial. He has a list of patients who are willing to testify that they were helped, even completely cured, by the treatment.

But once that first verdict has been handed down, nobody of any influence or authority will listen, or look at the evidence.

If the medical profession wants to find a cancer cure, why is it not willing to look for it wherever it might be? Are we to miss it because it originates in a small laboratory in the Southwest instead of the stainless steel and stone skyscraper of a multimillion-dollar research center?

Imagine if we had refused to use electricity because it was discovered by a publisher instead of a scientist, or refused to enjoy the Mona Lisa because it was painted by an inventor, instead of a full-time artist.

Closing

I have a few words to add. Medical practice has become a money making business these days. Expert Oncologists intentionally and knowingly use Radiation and Chemotherapy to kill people just to make money for making a better living for themselves. I would say it is a conspiracy against humanity. Genetic therapy was the biggest medical fraud of the 20th Century, and

Stem Cell therapy will be the biggest medical fraud of 21st Century.

Thank you for reading this book.

Autobiography

On April 24, 1915, my grandfather was arrested by the Ottoman Turkish soldiers and shot to death, just for being Armenian. He was a tobacco merchant and had nothing to do with politics. The same day my father picked up all family members and moved to Aleppo, Syria to avoid what happened to his father. My father could not find a job in Syria and returned to the Syrian-Turkish border to work in the train station on the Turkish side of the border. In 1916 my father married my mother, Marie Rezkalla Sadegh. In 1917 my brother Sarkis was born, and in 1918 my brother Taufic was born.

At that time the Turkish soldiers went door-to-door asking if any Armenians lived there. My mother told them in Arabic that no Armenians lived at that address.

At my mother's suggestion my father decided to change our name to an Arabic name to avoid harassment by the Turkish soldiers, so Chilkevorkian became Ashkar, which is the translation of Chil, which means red haired. Missal became Elias, Vartkes became Taufic.

However, changing the names to Arabic did not end the hassling. In 1919 a Turkish soldier who knew my father was at work decided to pick him up from the train station. In the evening the manager of the train station told my father to go home immediately and not to come back to work again because he was instructed to prepare all the Armenians working in the train station for pick up the next morning.

The next morning, when the soldiers could not find my father they asked the train station manager where my father was. The manager said that my father did not show up for work. They asked for my father's address so they could pick him up. Early in the morning, they knocked on my father's door as usual but this time they asked my mother by name where my father was, and since she realized that they knew exactly where my father lives, she could not lie to them and asked my father to come to face the soldiers.

The Turkish soldiers asked my father why he did not report to work and my father said that my older brother Sarkis was sick and he had to take him to the doctor. Luckily the soldiers told my father "Okay, take your child to the doctor and tomorrow morning we will come and pick you up at 9 o'clock." My father said he would report to work the next day, but the soldiers told him to not go to work and wait at home.

The Next day my father was ready, but it was 9:30 and nobody showed up. He then decided to go out to see why the soldiers did not come. When he opened the door, he saw the same two Turkish soldiers had been shot to death in front of his doorstep by advancing French soldiers.

Because of this, my father was so afraid that other Turkish soldiers may charge him for killing the Turkish soldiers, he decided to move the family to Beirut, Lebanon to start a new life far from the Turkish border.

In 1921 my third brother Antoine was born, in 1925 my sister Angel was born, and finally, on April 23, 1931, I was born.

I attended College of Saint Gregoire (a school) in Ashrafieh, Beirut, Lebanon.

On July 4, 1947, all of our family, except my sister, who was married, immigrated to Armenia in the Soviet Union and settled in the capital of Armenia, Yerevan.

From 1947 to 1952 I attended #44 school in Yerevan, Armenia.

In 1952 I graduated from high school and the same year was admitted to the physics faculty of the State University of Yerevan to study physics.

In 1956 I was at the Moscow State University for six months preparing to receive my graduation diploma in the field of cosmic rays from the physics department.

In 1957 I graduated University as a nuclear physicist, specializing in cosmic rays.

After graduation I was assigned to work in the cosmic laboratory of the same university as a senior researcher and was immediately sent to the city of Dubna, northwest of Moscow, to participate in research of the structure of matter at the International Research Center, using an electron accelerator (of course, it was only for the democratic country of eastern Europe).

After only two months in the laboratory, I was told to return home voluntarily or be fired. The reason was that I was denied clearance to work in the research center, which was considered secret. The basis for the denial of the clearance was: "unreliable foreign born citizen."

In 1959, to avoid constant denial of clearance to work in the secret nuclear research laboratories, I decided to move and start research in the mechanism polymerization of macromolecules, which was not considered a secret field. I got a position of senior researcher in VNISK, which was mainly involved in research and development of synthetic rubber, particularly Neoprene. Here also, involuntarily, I got involved in secret research for the Navy. This time the Navy needed to cover underwater torpedoes and mines with Neoprene rubber to avoid detection by sonar, an ultrasound detector, and I was the only person who could do the work because to do the job one needed knowledge in physics, and I was the only physicist. All other personnel consisted of chemical engineers. Work was completed successfully; still, I was denied access to see the results of the real test, which was conducted in the Baltic Sea by submarine. As a promotion, I was one of the eleven participants of the patent granted for that job and received 20.00 Rubles.

On September 12, 1959, I got married to Angel Jamil Khoukass, born on January 29, 1939, in Beirut, Lebanon (father Jamil, mother Azadouhi).

In 1962 I began studying for my doctorate in the Thermo-Chemical Laboratory at Moscow State University at Lomonosov, in Moscow.

In 1965, after finishing my doctorate in Chemical Physics, I got a position as senior researcher at the Physics Institute of Yerevan, in Armenia.

In 1965 I applied for an exit visa to immigrate back to my native country, Lebanon. After being denied many times, finally, six years later, in December 1970, I received my exit visa.

On March 12, 1971, I immigrated back to Lebanon, and on September 29, 1972, I and my wife entered the United States via J.F. Kennedy airport in New York City.

On June 21, 1977, I became an American citizen.

In the United States I first worked as an electrician, and in 1977 I was self-employed and actively making my research in cancer up-to-date.

In 1980 I found the cure for cancer. In 1983 I tested my cancer cure on a woman with breast cancer that had spread all over her body. Her recuperation was 100%.

In 1985 I was arrested and convicted as a criminal for finding a cure for cancer.

In 1990 I found a cure for HIV-AIDS, but I did not test it since I have no formal training to deal with a dangerous and contagious virus like HIV-AIDS.

In 1995 I had angioplasty surgery to place a stent in the artery of my heart.

In 1999 I had triple bypass heart surgery without any complications.

In 2003 I had pancreatic cancer and after five and a half hours of surgery five participating doctors told my wife to make funeral arrangements for me as they had no hope of saving my life. I immediately started the NIA treatment and saved my life.

In 2007, on Saturday, December 1, 2007, at 11:00 am my wife Angel passed away in New York City. She was 68 years old. She is resting at Forest Lawn Cemetery in Los Angeles, CA. (Note: My wife's blood pressure was high, and her doctor gave her blood pressure reducing medicine. She got brain damage and died later. My advice: Do not take a physician's recommended blood pressure reducing medicine.)

Bibliography

1. Daling JR, Madeleine MM, Johnson LG, et al. Penile cancer: the importance of circumcision, human papillomavirus and smoking in situ and invasive disease. IJC 2005; 116(4):60616.

2. Walboomers JMM, Jacobs MV, Manos MM. Human Papillomavirus is a necessary cause of invasive Cervical Cancer Worldwide. Journal of Pathology 1999(189):129.

3. Daling JR, Madeleine MM, Schwartz SM, et al. A population based study of squamous cell vaginal cancer: HPV and cofactors. Gynecol Oncol 2002; 84(2):26370.

4. Kagie MJ, Kenter GG, Zomerdijk Nooijen Y, et al.Human papillomavirus infection in squamous cell carcinoma of the vulva, in various synchronous epithelial changes and normal vulvar skin.

5. Daling JR, Madeleine MM, Johnson LG, et al. Human papillomavirus, smoking, and sexual practices in the etiology of anal cancer. Cancer 2004; 101(2): 27080.

6. Forman, D., Helicobacter pylori infection: a novel risk factor in the etiology of gastric cancer. J Natl Cancer Inst, 1991. 83(23): p. 17023.

7. Boshoff, C. and R. Weiss, AIDS related malignancies. Nat Rev Cancer, 2002. 2(5): p. 37382.

8. The Human Body, Bantam Books, 1971 USA

9. WOMAN'S BODY, Bantam Books, 1977. USA

10. UNDERSTANDING YOUR IMMUNE SYSTEM, Avon Books, 1986 USA

11. CancerHelp.UK For general information (http://cancerhelp.cancerresearchuk.org/)

I did not add any other articles because all articles since 1900 about the cure of cancer published in the leading medical journals such as New England Journal of Medicine, American Medical Association, Cancer, Lancet and much more are fraudulent and fake, so they do not deserve to be here to confuse people. All the articles in the medical journals about finding a cure for cancer should be shredded so as not to confuse other scientists involved in finding the cure for cancer.

Resources

Dr. George E. Ashkar's Website:
www.cancerselfcure.com, which includes Cancer Cure,
2010, by George E. Ashkar, Ph.D. and a video of how
to get started using his "Neutral Infection Absorption
(NIA) Treatment Method"

Below is a link to order *Cancer Cause and Cure: With
Mother and Daughter Stories of Removing Toxins with
Chickpeas*, 2017, by Bonnie O'Sullivan and Sandra
Petry and other books published by The Road To
Health Books:

https://roadtohealthbooks.com/

To follow Sandra (Sandy) Petry's continuing
experiences with her NIA treatment please go to:
Sandrastory.com